CALORIE DEFICIT PLAN BOOK
28 days journey to weightloss

By
Maria Escobar

Table of contents

INTRODUCTION

Welcome to the calorie deficit plan book In a world where health and fitness have become paramount, the Calorie Deficit Plan Book stands as your essential guide to achieving your weight management goals. This book is a comprehensive resource that will empower you with the knowledge and strategies to harness the power of calorie deficits to reach your desired level of fitness and well-being.

Whether you're looking to shed unwanted pounds, maintain a healthy weight, or simply better understand the science of nutrition and calorie balance, this book is designed to help you navigate the complex world of calories and their impact on your body. We'll break down the concept of a calorie deficit, explore its benefits, and provide you with practical, evidence-based advice on how to create and maintain a calorie deficit effectively.

Through expert insights, real-world success stories, meal planning tips, and exercise recommendations, the Calorie Deficit Plan Book will guide you on a journey towards a healthier, more vibrant you. Your path to a sustainable and balanced approach to nutrition and weight management begins here.

Are you ready to take control of your health and transform your life through the power of the calorie deficit? Let's embark on this enlightening and empowering journey together.

WHAT IS CALORIE DEFICIT

A calorie deficit is a fundamental concept in the realm of nutrition and weight management. It occurs when an individual consumes fewer calories through their diet than their body expends in daily activities and functions. In simpler terms, it means that you're taking in fewer calories than your body needs for maintenance and energy, resulting in a net reduction in your overall calorie intake.
A calorie deficit is a key principle for weight loss because, when you consistently maintain this deficit, your body starts to utilize its stored energy reserves, primarily in the form of body fat, to make up for the energy short-fall. This leads to a gradual reduction in body weight over time.

Creating a calorie deficit can be achieved through a combination of dietary changes (consuming fewer calories) and increased physical activity (burning more calories). It's an essential component of many weight loss and body recomposition strategies. However, it's important to create a calorie deficit in a healthy and sustainable manner to ensure long-term success and overall well-being. It's worth noting that individual calorie needs can vary based on factors like age, gender, activity level, and metabolism. Therefore, determining the appropriate calorie deficit for your goals and body is a personalized process and often best approached with guidance from a healthcare professional or registered dietitian.

How To Calculate Calories Deficiency

Calculating a calorie deficit involves understanding your current calorie intake and how many calories you need to consume to achieve your weight loss or maintenance goals. Here's a basic guideline on how to calculate it:

Determine your Basal Metabolic Rate (BMR): You can use the Harris-Benedict equation to estimate your BMR. The equation depends on your gender, age, weight, and height. These are the formulas for estimating BMR:

For Men: BMR = 88.362 + (13.397 × weight in kg) + (4.799 × height in cm) - (5.677 × age in years)

1. For Women: BMR = 447.593 + (9.247 × weight in kg) + (3.098 × height in cm) - (4.330 × age in years)
2. Calculate your Total Daily Energy Expenditure (TDEE): TDEE includes your BMR and the calories burned through physical activity. You can use a multiplier to estimate TDEE based on your activity level:
   - little or no exercise: BMR x 1.2

- light exercise or sports 1-3 days a week: BMR x 1.375
- moderate exercise or sports 3-5 days a week: BMR x 1.55
- hard exercise or sports 6-7 days a week: BMR x 1.725
- very hard exercise, physical job, or training twice a day: BMR x 1.9

3. Set your calorie intake goal: To lose weight, you generally need to consume fewer calories than your TDEE. The normal recommendation is to aim for a calorie deficit of 300 to 800 calories per day, which can lead to a safe and sustainable weight loss of about 1-2 pounds per week.

4. Track your daily calorie intake: Use a food diary or a calorie-tracking app to monitor your daily calorie

consumption. Ensure to record everything you eat and drink.

5. Monitor your progress: As you continue to track your calorie intake and maintain a calorie deficit, you can monitor your weight loss progress. It's very important I to be patient and consistent in your efforts.

- Remember that it's crucial to consult with a healthcare professional or a registered dietitian before starting any calorie-restricted diet to ensure it's safe and suitable for your individual needs and health goals.

Calorie Counting Process

Calorie counting is a method used to track your daily calorie intake. Here's a step-by-step process for calorie counting:

1. Set Your Goals:
   - Determine your fitness or weight goals, whether it's weight loss, maintenance, or muscle gain.
   - Calculate your daily calorie needs based on factors like age, gender, activity level, and goals.
2. Choose a Calorie Tracking Method:
   - Use a smartphone app, website, or pen and paper to record

your food and drink
consumption.

3. Read Nutrition Labels:

- Check the labels on
  packaged foods for
  information on
  calories, serving size,
  and macronutrients
  (carbohydrates,
  protein, and fat).

4. Weigh or Measure Your
    Food:

- Use a kitchen scale
  or measuring cups to
  accurately portion
  your food.

5. Record Everything:

- Log everything you
  eat and drink
  throughout the day,
  including snacks and
  condiments.

6. Be Accurate:

- Use portion sizes and
  measurements for
  accuracy.

- Avoid estimating too much, as it can lead to inaccuracies.

7. Track Beverages:
   - Don't forget to include calories from beverages like coffee, tea, and soda.

8. Monitor Serving Sizes:
   - Be mindful of portion sizes, as they greatly affect calorie intake.

9. Be Consistent:
   - Make calorie counting a daily habit to get an accurate picture of your consumption.

10. Adjust as Needed:
    - If you're not seeing progress toward your goals, consider adjusting your calorie intake and activity level.

11. Pay Attention to Macronutrients:

- Track not only total
  calories but also the
  breakdown of carbs,
  protein, and fat to
  ensure a balanced
  diet.

12. Avoid Obsession:

- Don't become overly
  obsessed with calorie
  counting, as it should
  be a tool to help you,
  not a source of
  anxiety.

13. Seek Professional
Guidance:

- If you have specific
  dietary needs or
  health concerns,
  consult a registered
  dietitian or healthcare
  professional.

14. Be Mindful of Quality:

- Focus on consuming
  nutrient-dense foods,
  as the quality of
  calories matters for
  your overall health.

15. Stay Hydrated:

- Ensure you're drinking enough water, which can also influence your appetite and overall health.

16. Regularly Review Your Progress:

- Assess your progress and make necessary adjustments to your calorie intake and diet plan.
- Remember, while calorie counting can be a useful tool for managing your diet, it's essential to prioritize the overall quality of your food choices and your overall health.

Create Calorie Deficit Method

Creating a calorie deficit is essential for weight loss.

Here are some methods to achieve it:

1. Reduce calorie intake: Consume fewer calories than your body burns by eating smaller portions, choosing lower-calorie foods, and avoiding high-calorie snacks and sugary drinks.
2. Count calories: Track your daily calorie intake using apps or food journals to ensure you stay within your calorie goals.
3. Increase physical activity: Burn more calories through exercise, such as cardio workouts, strength training, or simply being more active throughout the day.
4. Combine diet and exercise: A combination of reducing calorie intake and increasing physical activity can create a larger calorie deficit.
5. Choose nutrient-dense foods: Opt for foods that

provide essential nutrients
while being lower in calories
to help you feel full and
satisfied.

6. Eat smaller, more frequent
   meals: This can help control
   hunger and prevent
   overeating during meals.
7. Use portion control: to
   prevent overeating,pay
   attention to the size of your
   portion
8. Plan your meals: Preparing
   meals in advance can help
   you make healthier food
   choices and control your
   calorie intake.
9. Stay hydrated: Drinking
   water can help control
   hunger and prevent
   overeating.
10. Get enough sleep: Poor
    sleep can lead to
    overeating, so ensure you
    get adequate rest.

Remember, it's essential to create
a sustainable calorie deficit that
allows for gradual, healthy weight

loss, typically 1-2 pounds per week. Extreme calorie restriction can be harmful and is not recommended for long-term success. Consulting a healthcare professional or a registered dietitian is advisable before making significant changes to your diet and exercise routine.

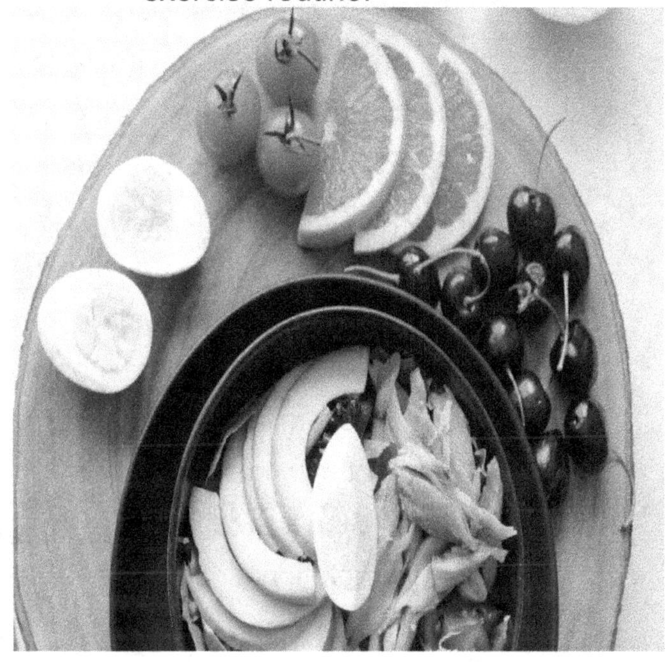

How to Consume few Calories

Certainly! Here are some tips on how to consume fewer calories:

1. Portion Control: Be mindful of serving sizes. Use smaller plates and bowls to help control portion sizs

2. Eat Slowly: Chew your food slowly and savor each bite.your body takes time to figure out when its full

3. Plan Meals: Prepare meals in advance and have healthy snacks readily available to reduce the temptation of high-calorie, convenient options.

4. Choose Water: Opt for water or other low-calorie beverages over sugary drinks, which can be high in empty calories.

5. Fill Up on Fiber: Include fiber-rich foods like fruits, vegetables, and whole grains in your diet. They can help you feel full and satisfied with fewer calories.

6. Avoid Processed Foods: Processed foods often contain hidden calories, added sugars, and unhealthy fats. Choose whole, unprocessed foods whenever possible.

7. Be Mindful of Sugar: Limit your intake of added sugars, as they can quickly add extra calories.Examine food labels to find hidden sources of sugar.

8. Limit Snacking: Try to stick to regular meal times and avoid excessive snacking between meals.

9. Cook at Home: When you cook at home, you have more control over the ingredients and can make healthier choices.

10. Track Your Intake: Consider keeping a food journal to monitor what you eat. You can become more anxious of your eating pattern by doing this.

11. Choose Lean Proteins: Opt for lean sources of protein like chicken, turkey, fish, and beans, as they are lower in calories and fat.

12. Opt for Grilled or Steamed: When dining out, choose grilled or steamed options instead of fried or heavily sauced dishes.

13. Control Temptations: Keep high-calorie, unhealthy foods out of your home to reduce the chances of indulging in them.

14. Get Plenty of Sleep: Lack of sleep can disrupt your hunger hormones and lead to overeating. Have at least 7-9 hours of quality sleep every night.

15. Stay Active: Regular physical activity can help you burn calories and maintain a healthy weight. Remember that it's essential to find an approach to reducing calorie intake that works for you and is sustainable in the long term. Consulting a healthcare professional or registered dietitian can also provide personalized guidance.

Calories in alcohol

- Alcohol contains calories, but the exact amount varies depending on the type of alcohol and its alcohol by volume (ABV) percentage. On average, a standard 1.5-ounce (44ml) shot of distilled spirits (like vodka, whiskey, or rum) contains approximately 96 calories. A 12-ounce (355ml) beer typically has around 150-200 calories, and a 5-ounce (148ml) glass of wine contains about 120-130 calories.

Keep in mind that mixers and additives in cocktails can significantly increase the calorie count. It's essential to be mindful of your alcohol consumption if you're trying to manage your calorie intake.

Reduce Highly Processed Food

- Reducing your intake of highly processed foods is a smart choice for your health. Here are some tips to help you achieve that:

1. Read Food Labels: Check the ingredient list for highly processed ingredients like refined sugars, trans fats, and artificial additives. Choose products with fewer and easily recognizable ingredients.
2. Cook at Home: Preparing meals at home allows you to control the ingredients and cooking methods, reducing

your reliance on packaged
and processed foods.

3. Choose Whole Foods: Opt
   for whole, unprocessed
   ingredients like fruits,
   vegetables, whole grains,
   and lean proteins. These
   foods are naturally nutritious
   and don't contain added
   chemicals.
4. Limit Sugary Drinks: Avoid
   sugary beverages like soda,
   energy drinks, and many
   fruit juices. Go for water,
   herbal tea, or normal water
   with no added sugars.
5. Snack Smart: Replace
   packaged snacks with
   healthier options like fresh
   fruit, nuts, yogurt, or
   homemade snacks like air-
   popped popcorn.
6. Reduce Fast Food: Limit
   your visits to fast-food
   restaurants, as their
   offerings are often highly
   processed and loaded with
   unhealthy ingredients.

7. Meal Planning: Plan your meals in advance and make a shopping list to avoid impulse purchases of processed foods.

8. Be Mindful of Sauces and Condiments: Many processed foods are hidden in condiments and sauces. Make your own or choose options with simple, recognizable ingredients.

9. Avoid Ready-Made Meals: Pre-packaged meals, frozen dinners, and instant noodles are typically high in processed ingredients. Cook fresh, whole meals instead.

10. Educate Yourself: Learn about the impact of highly processed foods on your health. Knowing and understanding the risks can motivate you to make healthy choices.

11. Gradual Changes: Transitioning to a less processed diet can be

challenging. Start by making small changes and gradually reduce your intake of processed foods.

12. Practice Moderation: It's okay to enjoy some processed treats occasionally, but moderation is key. Reserve them for special occasions rather than daily consumption.

13. Stay Informed: Keep updated on food and nutrition trends. As you gain more knowledge, you can make informed choices about the foods you consume.

Remember that reducing processed foods in your diet is a gradual process. Be patient with yourself and focus on making sustainable, long-term changes for a healthier lifestyle

Reduce processed food intake

Reducing the intake of highly processed foods is essential for maintaining a healthy diet. These foods often contain excessive sugar, salt, unhealthy fats, and additives. They lack essential nutrients and fiber while being calorie-dense. High consumption is linked to obesity, heart disease, and other health issues. Choosing whole, unprocessed foods like fruits, vegetables, lean proteins, and whole grains can promote better health and overall well-being.

Advantage of Home-Cooked Meals

Consuming home-cooked meals in a calorie deficit plan offers several advantages:

1. Portion Control: You have better control over portion sizes, making it easier to manage calorie intake.

2. Ingredient Selection: You can choose high-quality, nutritious ingredients and control added sugars, fats, and preservatives.

3. Customization: You can tailor recipes to your dietary needs, ensuring you get the right balance of macronutrients.

4. Reduced Hidden Calories: Home cooking minimizes hidden calories often found

in restaurant or processed foods.

5. Reduced Sodium: You can limit salt intake, which is often high in restaurant dishes.
6. Meal Planning: You can plan meals in advance, making it easier to stick to your calorie deficit goals.
7. Freshness: Home-cooked meals are often fresher and contain more nutrients than pre-packaged options.
8. Cost-Efficiency: Cooking at home can be more budget-friendly than dining out or ordering takeout.
9. Skill Development: It's an opportunity to develop cooking skills and a deeper understanding of nutrition.
10. Long-Term Sustainability: Home cooking can be a sustainable and healthier approach to maintaining a calorie deficit over time.

Calorie Deficit Food Plan List

- Creating a calorie deficit food plan involves consuming fewer calories than your body needs to maintain its current weight. Here's a list of foods to include in such a plan:

1. Lean Proteins:
   - Chicken breast
   - Turkey
   - Fish (salmon, tilapia, cod)
   - Lean cuts of beef or pork
   - Tofu
   - Greek yogurt

2. Vegetables:
   - Leafy greens (spinach, kale, lettuce)
   - Broccoli
   - Cauliflower

- Bell peppers
- Carrots
- Zucchini

3. Fruits:
   - Berries (strawberries, blueberries, raspberries)
   - Apples
   - Oranges
   - Grapefruit
   - Bananas (in moderation)

4. Whole Grains:
   - Brown rice
   - Quinoa
   - Oats
   - Whole wheat pasta
   - Barley

5. Legumes:
   - Lentils
   - Chickpeas
   - Black beans
   - Kidney beans

6. Nuts and Seeds (in moderation):
   - Almonds
   - Walnuts
   - Chia seeds

- Flaxseeds

7. Dairy (low-fat or non-fat):
   - Milk
   - Yogurt
   - Cheese

8. Healthy Fats:
   - Avocado
   - Olive oil
   - Coconut oil (in moderation)

9. Snacks (in moderation):
   - Hummus with veggies
   - Greek yogurt with honey
   - Air-popped popcorn

10. Beverages:
    - Water
    - Green tea
    - Herbal tea
    - Black coffee (without added sugar)
      Remember to portion control and monitor your daily calorie intake to ensure you maintain a calorie deficit.

Avoid These Calorie-Dense Food

While on a calorie deficit plan, it's important to be mindful of your food choices and focus on foods that provide essential nutrients without excessive calories. Here are some foods to avoid or limit:

1. Sugary Snacks: Avoid candies, cookies, cakes, and sugary beverages as they are high in empty calories.

2. Fried Foods: Limit deep-fried items like French fries, fried chicken, and potato chips, as they are high in unhealthy fats.

3. Sugary Drinks: Cut back on soda, fruit juices, and energy drinks, which can be

calorie-dense and lack nutritional value.
4. Processed Foods: Reduce consumption of highly processed foods, like fast food, frozen meals, and packaged snacks, which often contain hidden calories.
5. High-Fat Dairy: Opt for low-fat or fat-free dairy products to reduce calorie intake.
6. White Bread and Pasta: Choose whole grains over refined grains for better satiety and nutrient content.
7. High-Calorie Sauces: Be cautious with creamy, cheesy, or sugary sauces and dressings used in dishes.
8. Alcohol: Alcohol contains empty calories and can lower inhibitions, leading to overeating.

Instead, focus on lean proteins, vegetables, fruits, whole grains, and foods that are rich in nutrients but lower in calories to help you stay on track with your calorie deficit plan.

Weight Loss Tips.

Certainly! Here are some weight loss success tips:

1. Set Realistic Goals: Start with achievable and realistic weight loss goals to avoid frustration.

2. Balanced Diet: Focus on a balanced diet with plenty of fruits, vegetables, lean proteins, and whole grains.

3. Portion Control: Be mindful of portion sizes to avoid overfeeding.

4. Stay Hydrated: Drink plenty of water to help control appetite and stay hydrated.

5. Regular Exercise: Ensure regular physical activity into your routine, combining cardio and strength training.

6. Monitor Your Progress: Keep a food journal or use apps to track your eating habits and workouts.

7. Get Adequate Sleep: Aim for 7-9 hours of quality sleep to support your weight loss efforts.

8. Manage Stress: Find suitable ways to cope with stress to prevent emotional eating.

9. Seek Support: Consider joining a weight loss group or talking to a healthcare professional for guidance and support.

10. Be Patient: Weight loss takes time; be patient and persistent in your efforts. Remember, what works for one person may not work for another, so it's important to find a strategy that suits your individual needs and preferences.

Track Calorie Intake

Keeping track of your calorie intake is an important aspect of maintaining a healthy diet and managing your weight. Here are some key points to consider:

1. Understanding Caloric Needs: Start by determining your daily caloric needs based on factors like age, gender, activity level, and weight goals. This can be done using online calculators or consulting with a nutritionist.

2. Record Your Intake: Keep a food diary or use a calorie tracking app to log everything you eat and drink. Be thorough and accurate, including portion sizes.

3. Read Nutrition Labels: Pay attention to nutrition labels

on packaged foods to know
the calorie content of each
item. This helps you make
informed choices.

4. Portion Control: Be mindful
   of portion sizes to avoid
   overeating. Measuring your
   food can be helpful in this
   regard.

5. Stay Consistent: Try to be
   consistent with your tracking
   to get a more accurate
   picture of your daily calorie
   intake over time.

6. Monitor Progress: Regularly
   assess your progress and
   make adjustments as
   needed to meet your health
   and fitness goals.

7. Quality Matters: While
   calorie counting is
   important, don't forget the
   quality of the calories you
   consume. Aim for a
   balanced diet with a variety
   of nutrients, including
   proteins, carbohydrates, and
   healthy fats.

8. Seek Professional
    Guidance: If you have
    specific dietary or health
    goals, consider consulting a
    registered dietitian or
    nutritionist for personalized
    advice and support.
    Remember that calorie
    counting is just one aspect
    of a healthy diet. It's
    essential to focus on overall
    nutrition and make
    sustainable lifestyle
    changes for long-term
    health and well-being.

Consume whole food

Consuming whole foods is a
healthy choice, as they are
minimally processed and
retain their natural nutrients.
Fruits, vegetables, whole
grains, lean proteins, and
nuts are great examples of
whole foods.

Increase Activity Level

- Increasing your activity level is a great way to improve your overall health. You can start by incorporating regular exercise into your routine.
- such as walking, jogging, swimming, or other activities you enjoy. Additionally, consider making small changes in your daily life, like taking the stairs instead of the elevator, or parking farther from your destination to get more steps in. It's important to find activities that you enjoy, as it'll make it easier to stick with a more active lifestyle.

Don't Stress About Weight

It's important not to stress about your weight. Focus on

maintaining a normal and healthy lifestyle through balanced nutrition and daily exercise. Your self-worth is not determined by your weight, and it's essential to prioritize mental and emotional well-being

Summary

A 28-day weight loss plan is a structured program designed to help individuals lose weight in a healthy and sustainable way over the course of four weeks. These plans typically include a combination of balanced diet, regular exercise, and lifestyle changes. The specifics can vary, but the main goal is to create a calorie deficit to promote fat loss while

maintaining
nutritional balance
and promoting long-
term habits. It's
important to consult
with a healthcare
professional before
starting any weight
loss plan to ensure
it's safe and suitable
for your individual
needs and health
status